DAVID SMALLEY

Me and Uncle Arthur:
a Story of Arthritis

Published by

MELROSE BOOKS

An Imprint of Melrose Press Limited
St Thomas Place, Ely
Cambridgeshire
CB7 4GG, UK
www.melrosebooks.com

FIRST EDITION

Copyright © David Smalley 2008

The Author asserts his moral right to
be identified as the author of this work

Cover designed by Jeremy Kay

ISBN 978-1-906050-91-7

All rights reserved. No part of this publication may be reproduced, stored in a retrieval system, or transmitted, in any form or by any means electronic, mechanical, photocopying, recording or otherwise, without the prior permission of the publishers.

This book is sold subject to the condition that it shall not, by way of trade or otherwise, be lent, re-sold, hired out or otherwise circulated without the publisher's prior consent in any form of binding or cover other than that in which it is published and without a similar condition including this condition being imposed on the subsequent purchaser.

Printed and bound in Great Britain by:
CPI Antony Rowe, Chippenham, Wiltshire

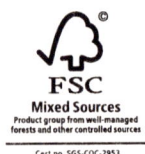

CONTENTS

Introduction v
1 – Introducing Uncle Arthur 1
2 – The Weather, Food and Drink 3
3 – Frustration and Embarrassment 9
4 – A Daydream and Another Bad Day 20
5 – The Arguments with Uncle Arthur 24
6 – The Marathon 30
7 – Symptoms 39
8 – Children and the Elderly 42
9 – The Friendly Chat with Uncle Arthur 45
10 – The Dream Day Uncle Arthur Grants Me 54
11 – Birthdays, Christmas and Anniversaries 64
12 – The Trench 78
13 – A Brief Summary 80
14 – Present Day 82

INTRODUCTION

This book tells of the ups and downs of an Arthritis sufferer, from the embarrassing, sad and depressing moments with the illness to the rare triumphs against all the odds. My story takes you on my own personal journey so far, and is told over the twelve months leading up to my tenth anniversary as an Arthritis sufferer. To this day Arthritis is still very much linked to older people even though it affects many children and younger people worldwide, and is still a very dark and un-talked-about subject. Therefore my aim is to raise general awareness of this dreadful problem.

The story takes you on a roller coaster ride between the two characters, which are myself and my Uncle Arthur, which is my Arthritis. The two characters strike up an unlikely bond as they pit their wits and emotions against each other. My story is a light-hearted account of a very serious subject, with the two characters trying to out-manoeuvre each other on the battlefield – the battlefield being everyday life for the Arthritis sufferer.

Chapter One

INTRODUCING UNCLE ARTHUR

This is a story about my Uncle Arthur and me. He's quite a character, as you will see. I've not always known my Uncle Arthur, in fact I have only known him for nine years, but please trust me – that's damned long enough. You see he's not your typical Uncle, he's not the sort that buys you presents and looks after you, and he's not the sort that takes you down the pub for a pint when you turn eighteen, and he isn't the sort that even loves you, oh no he is certainly none of them. In fact he is just a bastard who likes to bring pain and misery into my life.

We have many fights and arguments because we never see eye-to-eye with each other. He is a dark and gloomy chap who doesn't let people know too much about him, you could say he operates in mysterious ways.

My Uncle Arthur is both a bully and a coward because he hides and attacks me when I am feeling vulnerable and at a low.

Think of a really bad character in a film, someone who is evil, dark and sad – that would be my Uncle Arthur.

He would play the bad character and I would play the good guy, but unlike in the films the good guy won't win this one, I won't be Gary Cooper in High Noon or Clint Eastwood in *The Good, The Bad, And The Ugly*, because not even a six-shooter can kill this bad guy.

You see, no matter how many fights and battles you have with him he will always want to win. I sometimes wish I was dreaming all this and that I was just in a film, but I am not, I fight with him every day; it seems strange to say you fight with your Uncle every day but it's true, I do.

Have you ever met someone you wish you hadn't?

I suppose everybody has. I hate the day I met Uncle Arthur, I knew from the very first moment he came into my life that I wouldn't like him. He first shook me by my right hand, and that is where he has stayed ever since, only now he occupies both hands. As if that's not bad enough the cheeky swine now occupies my right foot. If he tries moving into my left foot I will kick him right between the legs. The fact that he has decided to travel with me makes my life different in many ways.

Chapter Two

THE WEATHER, FOOD AND DRINK

Having an Uncle like this means I can't do some of the things people take for granted in everyday life. I will come to some of those things later. I wish I could just drop him off at some roadside or throw him off a bridge somewhere, but I can't: for the time being I am stuck with him. At least he doesn't snore – I suppose that's one thing to be grateful for. In fact when he's asleep he doesn't bother me too much, he doesn't nag me, he just lets me lead my own life, which is great. I just wish he would sleep more often than he does. It's funny, he always seems to go to sleep when it's warm weather. If only I could get him to sleep when it's cold and damp and wet because that's when he's at his grumpiest. During these sorts of weather conditions he can be really nasty with me and this is when he decides to hurt me the most.

I don't know what it is but he seems to know when it is going to be damp or rainy. I haven't really worked him out yet, but somehow he seems to know what the weather is going to be like before I do. Maybe he has psychic powers? If so, I wish he would put them to better use and predict the lotto numbers or back me a winner on the horses instead of giving me all this grief when it turns out to be cold and damp.

The weather causes a lot of the fights me and Uncle Arthur have. If it's sunny I will just give him a slap round the head and tell him to go and bug somebody else, and that usually works because he knows that when it's warm weather he can't hurt me as much as he would like to.

But when it's cold and damp he comes at me with all guns blazing, and no matter how many times I slap him round the head and tell him to go away he just doesn't listen, he just uses my body as some sort of punch bag and seems to get a kick out of beating me up. The sad thing is when it rains or when it's cold, I can't do anything to stop him and he knows it. The defences in my body help me cope with him better when it's warm, but there is nothing I can really do to stop him when it's damp and cold.

The only way I can calm him down is to take him down the local pub and get him drunk. The more I drink the less he seems to nag me, the beer just drowns him out. Now this is all fine and dandy but it's costing me a bloody fortune. There must be other ways to get rid of him?

I used to give him drugs to shut him up. They worked for a while but when he woke up he was like a bear with a sore head. He would be in a terrible mood and have a right go at me – sometimes he would beat me up for the next couple of days, so I stopped giving him the drugs as they were just fuelling his already bad temper. I wish I could take him on holiday more, somewhere really warm where he can lie on a beach and sleep his hangovers off, but I just can't afford it and I can't really rely on our weather, can I? So you see I am stuck with him.

Uncle Arthur is not someone you can just send to some sort of rehab centre or top-notch hospital because as yet nobody has found a cure for him, and if no one has found a cure for him yet, what's the point in sending him there in the first place? I might as well save my bus fare and buy a bag of chips or something – but don't tell Uncle Arthur I am buying chips because he doesn't like me eating them, especially the greasy ones. I suppose this brings me nicely onto the subject of food.

Uncle Arthur must be the fussiest person in the world when it comes to food. You see, food causes a lot of the fights that we have. He is so crafty you wouldn't believe it. He makes me think that he doesn't mind what I feed him; he says yes I don't mind that, and I don't mind this, and I can drink this, and I can drink that.

Here is a classic example of what I mean. I will say to him, 'What do you fancy to eat tonight Uncle Arthur?' Now if it happens to be a Monday he will ask for a kebab with all the trimmings, so I buy him a kebab with everything on it. Now he will normally sit at the bar in the local pub with me and scoff it all down, with a bag of chips thrown in for good measure. He will then wash it all down with five or six pints of lager. Now for the rest of the night he will be in a really good mood after his little feast, especially when he knows I have paid for it. He never says thank you or kiss my arse, he just sits there burping like a bloated pig.

At the end of the night he will get up, say his goodbyes and trundle off home, and that's a typical Monday night for him. He always comes across as though he has really enjoyed his night out, which is great for me because he leaves me alone and doesn't bother me. On the whole he just lets me enjoy my night, which is great. So there you have it, a good night had by all.

But when he wakes up on Tuesday morning he proves to me once again what a complete and utter ungrateful git he is. Instead of waking me up in the morning nice and bonny and letting me look forward to the day ahead, he wakes me up with a lot of pain all over my body – well, the parts of my body where he decides to sleep. When I ask him why he is causing me this pain after such a good night out, the cheeky sod tells me it's the food he has eaten and the lager he drank the night before. So

I ask him why he is blaming me for his anger? He then shouts back at the top of his voice that it was my fault, that I had filled him with all that bad food and drink and that I should be more responsible, being the owner of the body in which he sleeps. He says, 'You had no right filling me with lager and kebabs.'

I say, 'Why not, you were having a good night weren't you?'

'No, you were having a good night and you just assumed I was too. You know that sort of food and drink aggravates me, you know it makes me feel really rough – and you know what that means? If I feel really rough then you are going to feel really rough too.'

'Well,' I say, 'why didn't you say something to me when we were sat at the bar?'

'I didn't say anything because I wanted to see if you had learned your lesson from the previous times when you filled me with lager and kebabs. You know I always wake up in a bad mood when you have eaten things like that.'

I say, 'Well I like kebabs and lager.'

He replies, 'I don't care whether you like lager and kebabs because this is not about you; it's about me.'

So I say to him, 'What am I supposed to do when all my mates at the bar are drinking lager and eating kebabs – just sit there and watch them?'

'You should have gone hungry, and if you didn't want to go hungry you should have ordered something else.'

'Like what?' I say.

'Where do you want me to start? You know the foods I like, and you know the foods I dislike, and you know the foods which keep me quiet, and you know the foods which make me angry.'

'Yes, I know the foods you like; I know you want fresh fish with loads of oil in it or fresh chicken and vegetables.'

Then in a cocky manner he says, 'Well, if you know what I want why don't you give them to me? What was stopping you giving the kebab shop a miss for a change and cooking something really healthy for us when we got home?'

'Do you really think I'm going to go home and cook you something when I've had a few pints? I'd burn the bloody house down,' I reply angrily.

That's what upsets me about him, it's okay when he's sitting there scoffing his face out and swilling his lager and basically having a free night, but when he wakes up in the morning with a hangover and bad guts he takes it out on me. Now this really upsets me so there's only one thing for it – no more kebabs for him. As a matter of fact I have a good mind to keep the lager away from him as well. Maybe that's a bit harsh, maybe I am over reacting a bit with the lager. I don't know.

I will have to see whether he treats me any better over the next couple of days.

Chapter Three

FRUSTRATION AND EMBARRASSMENT

It's funny, I even had my doctor scratching his head the other day. I went to him because Uncle Arthur was really playing me up and I was hoping the doctor could give him something to calm him down. Anyway, I went in and said, 'Hello doctor, I'd like you to help me.'

'What can I do for you?' he replied.

I said I wanted him to kill my Uncle Arthur. Well, he gave me a funny look and said, 'I am a doctor, not a murderer.'

I said, 'No, you don't understand.' Again I found myself explaining to someone that my Uncle Arthur was not a real Uncle.

He looked a little puzzled and said, 'I don't understand.'

'No, of course you don't understand,' I said. 'You

see, he's not real … well, he is real – what I mean is he's not a real Uncle, I just pretend he's my Uncle.' At this stage the doctor asked if I was sure there was nothing else he could prescribe me.

I think he wanted to give me something for the state of my mental health. At that point I felt it better to explain that my Uncle Arthur is my Arthritis.

'Oh,' he said, still looking really puzzled. 'Why do you call your Arthritis Uncle Arthur?' he asked.

Now that was a rather good question, which put me on the spot. I realised then that I didn't really know why I called him Uncle Arthur, I suppose it just sounds better than the dark and gloomy word of Arthritis. Anyway my eventual answer was, 'I don't know.'

'Fine,' he said. 'Now let's talk about your Arthritis … or your Uncle Arthur as you call it.'

I gave the doctor a brief description of what my Uncle Arthur was like and told him about the way he had treated me over the years.

He seemed to understand, and started to build my hopes up. I got a little excited, thinking he was going to put an end to my troubles in some way. But my hopes were soon dashed. As soon as I saw him reach for his prescription book, I realised my hopes for some help or for some miraculous cure were not going to be fulfilled. I knew he just wanted to give Uncle Arthur some of those drugs which make him sleep for a while. So I told the doctor I didn't want to take the drugs.

'Why not?' he said.

So I said to him, 'You don't understand, you just don't understand. What you doctors don't realise is that when you give someone like my Uncle Arthur these sort of things, after a while when the effects of the drugs wear off he will turn really angry with me and cause me even more pain.'

The doctor said, 'Well, why have you come here in the first place if you don't want the drugs?'

He was right. I don't know why I went, I guess I knew deep down what the outcome would be, maybe I went because it's a cry for help? I don't know. I thought that if my Uncle Arthur knew I was trying to help him he wouldn't get so angry with me and maybe he would leave me alone for a while, but that's just living in hope because it won't happen. So my long and lonely battle with Uncle Arthur continues; when will it end?

There are many reasons why society doesn't know much about the likes of my Uncle Arthur. There are many questions still unanswered about him. Like for example, why do certain foods set him off? And why do certain types of weather conditions arouse his hormones, and why does he like to attack the joints? Why doesn't he attack other parts of the body where he would have more to feed on, like a flabby belly or a wobbly arse? When he arrives at the joints I am sure he thinks he is sitting down to his Sunday roast. I bet he thinks he is sitting down to a nice joint of lamb or something. When he is dining on my joints and sucking all the vital juices from them, I sometimes feel like shouting down to him: 'Excuse me, would you like some of that nice mint sauce to go with my joints?' Do you remember that famous quote from the Humphrey Bogart film *Casablanca*: 'Of all the gin joints in all of the world; she had to walk into mine.' Well that's how I feel: of all the human bodies in all of the world, Uncle Arthur had to walk into mine.

When you are fighting Arthritis – or Uncle Arthur – you're not only fighting him; you are not only fighting the pain and humiliation that he brings on a daily basis, you are fighting something far worse. You are fighting Stress. Stress is an old friend of Uncle Arthur's and sometimes he decides to come and visit. Sometimes his visits are short, but sometimes he will come for a couple of weeks, or even months. The problem is that when he comes to visit Uncle Arthur he is visiting me at the same time. When Stress comes to visit, it affects me quite badly because it makes me feel sad and lonely and I start to get depressed with everything. I seem to lose all sense of direction and purpose and I sometimes feel I am losing the will to battle on through my illness. I am quite a strong and determined type of chap, but that doesn't stop me from shedding tears of sadness from time to time.

The one thing I always have to tell myself is that whilst I live with my Uncle Arthur a cloud called depression will always loom over me, but I must be strong. I have got to be strong because if I am not, between them

Uncle Arthur and his mate Stress will eventually kill me off. They will kill my mind first and then my body, but I mustn't let them. I must stand up to them and if they knock me down I should just get back up and dust myself off.

Do you know the best way I can get at my Uncle Arthur? Well it's simple – I just laugh at him. When I laugh at him he doesn't like it, he wonders why I am laughing when he is causing me so much pain. You see, some of the things he does to me make me laugh, he doesn't know it but they do. It's some of the cheeky things he does to me that just make me chuckle. He sometimes tries to embarrass me when people are watching; he tries to show me up in front of them. Let me give you an example.

The other day I went to a barbecue with some friends. When we got there the host shoved a beefburger under my nose and said, 'Here, get that down you.' Well you can't go to a Barbie and not have a beefburger so I scoffed it down as I was starving. So far so good.

At that point the host said, 'Here, wash that burger down with that.' It was a can of lager. 'Cheers,' I said, and that's when the fun started with my Uncle Arthur. The clever swine wouldn't let me open the can in front of anybody – every time I tried to pull the ring-pull back he shot terrible pains through my fingers and it made it worse because the ring-pull on the can was really tight, as they sometimes are. By this time all my mates had cracked open their cans and were guzzling the lager down, but not me, I was just standing there like a right pillock unable to open my can. So I said, 'Come on Uncle Arthur, the fun is over, let me open my can.'

He said, 'No, I am not going to let you open the can on your own, I am going to embarrass you in front of all your mates.'

I knew what he wanted me to do: he wanted me to ask one of my mates to open the can for me, knowing they would probably laugh at me. I tried to open it with the other hand but he wouldn't let me.

At that point I just laughed, as I could kind of see the funny side of what he was up to. Anyway, not to be outdone by him I decided to open the can with my house key, out of the sight of my mates. You see, the clever sod has no answer to house keys, and as I drank the lager I started to laugh at him as I had turned the joke around on him.

I could tell he wasn't best pleased, but sod him, I was dying of thirst.

Anyway, embarrassment did eventually catch up with me. One of the girls at the Barbie – whom I quite fancied – came up to me. I didn't know her, she was a friend of a friend. She said, 'Excuse me, why have you got such fat fingers? Why are they so fat? And why are you limping when you walk?'

Well, what could I say to that? At first I thought of saying I was a professional footballer and that I had picked up an injury during a match, and as for my fat fingers I was going to say I did a bit of boxing and that they had swelled up during a bout I had the night before. Now I suppose this would make me look quite macho and maybe impress the girl. But instead of seizing my chance, I completely blew it. I just came out with a load of old claptrap. I said, 'It's my Uncle Arthur, he doesn't like burgers and lager because they bloat him up.' What an absolutely daft answer that was, but it was the first thing that came into my head.

'Uncle Arthur?' she said. 'Who's Uncle Arthur?'

Good question, I thought. I probably could have explained, but I didn't, because for some strange reason I felt embarrassed, and that's why I came out with such a daft answer. At that point somebody interrupted her and so the conversation changed. I was really annoyed with myself, not because the conversation hadn't gone that well, but because I had let Uncle Arthur get the better of me. I was annoyed because I let the embarrassment of having Arthritis get the better of me, because my immediate thought was that if the girl knew I had Arthritis she wouldn't want to go out with me, and that's the wrong thing to think. I was really shocked that she had noticed how swollen my fingers were, and I wasn't expecting her to say what she said. I was hoping she might have said, 'Hello handsome, do you fancy a shag?'

Well, just because I have Arthritis it doesn't mean I can't dream a little.

Now, the example of him not letting me open my can of lager without giving me pain to my hands and fingers, is his way of trying to annoy me and embarrass me in front of other people, but most of the time he tries to annoy or embarrass me when nobody is there, just him and me.

Let me give you another example. Something really embarrassing happened to me the other day: even though it wasn't funny at the time, I have laughed to myself about it since. I had to ring my work to say I was going to be late – in fact I was going to be very late. When I got through to my boss and told him, he said okay and then asked me why. Now this was where the embarrassment started for me again. I have always been very honest, so I had to be honest again. I said to my boss that I couldn't get out of the door. He laughed and said, 'Why, have you forgotten where it is?' At this point I found his humour a little annoying. I knew that if I could explain this one away I could explain my way out of anything, so I said, 'I can't undo the door.'

'What do you mean?' he asked. 'Have you lost your key?'

'No, I haven't lost my key, I just can't open the door,' I replied.

'Well, why can't you open the door?' he asked.

So I told him the frost had come down last night and with the doors being wooden they had swelled up and jammed.

You see, when the doors jam like that Uncle Arthur won't let me open them. When I try and apply pressure to the door handle he says oh no you don't and shoots those agonising pains through my hands and fingers, which makes me let go. He literally traps me in my own home. The more I try to open the door, the more he hurts me.

So I have no choice but to wait for the frost to melt, which will give me a better chance of opening the door.

When the doors are not jammed Uncle Arthur normally lets me out without giving me too much grief. Don't get me wrong – he still lets me know he's there, but at least he lets me out of the house. It's like him saying a little good morning to me. Now, you can imagine what it was like trying to explain to my boss that I couldn't get out of the house because my Uncle Arthur wouldn't let me. He would probably assume that I was still drunk from the night before, so I calmly told him that it was my Arthritis that was playing me up and explained to him that I couldn't grip the door handles hard enough to open them.

I knew what he was thinking: I was trying to pull a fast one. I knew he wouldn't understand what I was talking about, why would he?

This is the sort of humiliation Uncle Arthur throws at me. I am thirty-six years old and I can't even get out of my own house when we've had frost the night before. Well, it's a great life I am having, I am loving every bloody minute of it.

I'm sorry for swearing. I just get a little upset with everything sometimes. People with an illness like mine will often feel this frustration and anger. Just when we think we are coping with the problem, the illness will often remind us that we are not. This frustration often turns to anger, and like everybody else we have to let off some steam.

But there is often something that will make us dig deep and carry on the battle with it – mine is the thought of others who are worse off than me. I sometimes feel I am climbing a never-ending mountain, but I know that others are climbing bigger and tougher mountains than mine. When I think of some of the things people face in their lives it sort of makes me think that my Uncle Arthur isn't that bad after all. Don't get me wrong – he will always be a nuisance, but he's not as bad as some of the nasty things other people have to carry round with them on a daily basis. At least I can eat and drink when I want; even if Uncle Arthur doesn't always agree with what I eat and drink, the point is I can still do it. There are some people in the world who don't know where their next meal is coming from and that saddens me: it should sadden everyone; even somebody as hardfaced as my Uncle Arthur should be saddened by the plight of some people. I can wear nice clothes – that's one thing Uncle Arthur can't deny me. Alright, he might be a swine and not let me fasten a tight button on my shirt, or he might not let me fasten my shoelaces properly, but I can live with that because there are some people in the world who have to wear rags for clothes, the same rags day in and day out, and that saddens me too. A lump comes to my throat when I think of the people who are blinded from birth, they have never seen the simple things in life that we take for granted, like the sunset and sunrise, and the moon and the stars, they have never seen the smiles on people's faces or the tears that roll from their eyes.

You see, why should I moan, why should any of us moan? There is a true saying in life, a very true saying: there is always somebody worse off than ourselves, and so to think of these people should make us stronger in our own plight.

Chapter Four

A DAYDREAM AND ANOTHER BAD DAY

The other day I was sitting thinking to myself and a great thought came into my mind. If I could spend one day without my Uncle Arthur, what would I do and where would I go? Now that is a good question.

This would be the day I would wish for. I would get up early in the morning without the pain I normally have, I would then have the biggest fry-up the world has ever seen. Then I would go upstairs and clean my teeth, not having to worry about the pain from trying to squeeze the last bit of toothpaste out of an almost empty tube.

Then I would get dressed, this time fastening all the buttons on my shirt and therefore looking a bit smarter for a change. Then I would put my shoes on and tie the laces properly – so much so that I wouldn't have to keep re-tying them every ten minutes like I normally do. One of the things I've really missed since my Uncle Arthur arrived is a good game of golf. (A lot of people say that a game of golf is a long walk spoiled. I don't really agree with them but they are entitled to their own opinion.)

I have always enjoyed playing golf because I find it so relaxing. Okay, the game might be a swine to play sometimes, as everybody who plays it will tell you, but no matter how many worries you have in life they just seem to disappear when you're playing golf. I don't know what it is, maybe it's because it's so tranquil and quiet? Maybe it's because some of the courses are so beautiful with the greenery and the trees? It just seems to take you away from the everyday hustle and bustle of life. So it would be great to get a few mates together and go for a good old round of golf. It would be great to be able to grip the clubs again and remind my mates how good I am. After winning the game by at least five shots, I would then throw a massive party at night for everyone.

Apart from having a few drinks in peace and not having to worry about how my Uncle Arthur would be feeling in the morning, there is one other thing I would really enjoy from the night. When you go to parties everyone shakes hands and stuff, either because they haven't seen each other for a while or because they are just generally glad to be there and having a good time. Now shaking hands for most people is normal, but for me it is usually a nightmare. You see, because Uncle

Arthur sleeps in my hands, when people grip my hand and squeeze it Uncle Arthur thinks they are trying to throttle him, so he reacts in the same way as anyone else would when they think they are being attacked: he shoots these horrible pains down my hands as if to say tell your mate not to come near me again. Now I could probably handle this pain or gesture from Uncle Arthur if it only happened once, but when there are hundreds of people at a party ... well, you can imagine, so being free to shake people's hands without worrying about the consequences would be great.

Now, the sort of day I have just talked about would seem a simple and normal day to most people, and rightly so, but to me it would be a really special day. Anyway, for now I will just have to keep wishing for that day. Only Uncle Arthur will decide when I can have days like that. Maybe they will always be a thing of the past – I don't know.

Today hasn't been the best of days for me. I seem to have been struggling with everything. This morning I couldn't squeeze the last bit of toothpaste from my tube and so I set out with smelly breath. Then at lunchtime I bought some dinner and couldn't open the screw top on the pop bottle I had bought – why manufacturers have to put those tops on so tight I don't know. The only way I could open it was to put the top in the door and use the door as a lever. This worked but because I had been wrestling with the bottle, the gases inside had built up, so when the top finally came off, the pop spurted out all over me and wet me through. The things you have to do to get a drink of pop.

Then this afternoon I went to put some petrol in my car, but I couldn't squeeze the pump hard enough to get the petrol in. I was going to ask the attendant to help me but again my pride got in the way and so I struggled, using both hands. That just about worked, but when you use both hands on the nozzle, you have less control over it, and because of this I ended up putting more petrol in than I wanted. I was only going to put five pounds in because that's all I had on me, but I squeezed too hard and ended up putting five pounds six pence in. I had to go into the shop and explain to the man behind the counter. He was kind enough to let the six pence go, so I thanked him and said it wouldn't happen again, knowing deep down that it probably would happen again. The only thing I can do next time is take more money with me than I need.

And to round off my crap day, I forgot my dental appointment. So there you have more examples of me struggling with basic day-to-day things thanks to my Arthritis, some in private and some in public. Because I have had a bad day, I am going down to the pub in the hope of getting drunk. Getting drunk is something I seem to be doing quite a lot of these days as my ups and downs continue.

Chapter Five

THE ARGUMENTS WITH UNCLE ARTHUR

In the morning Uncle Arthur was sitting there waiting for me as usual. There was a silence for a while. Then he said to me, 'You have no will-power.'

'What do you mean, I have no will-power?'

'You just haven't,' he said back to me.

'Yes I have,' I replied.

'If you had will-power you wouldn't be drinking the way you do,' he told me.

'Yes, well it's none of your business what I drink!' I shouted back at him.

'When you drink like you do, you make it my business,' he replied.

Deep down I knew he was right, but I couldn't admit it to him. At that point I couldn't work out whether Uncle Arthur actually did care for me after all and was just trying to warn me off the alcohol? But what he said next proved to me he didn't care about me at all. He called me an idiot.

'Why have you just called me an idiot?' I asked him. He said I was an idiot because I had wasted my chance with that girl at the barbecue. 'What's she got to do with my so-called drinking problem, and why have you suddenly brought her up?'

'Because you haven't been the same since that barbecue,' he replied.

'What do you mean, I haven't been the same?'

'You've been walking round for the last couple of days with a face that looks like a slapped arse.'

'Well, maybe it's because I'm just fed up with you bugging me every day?'

'No, I can definitely tell when you're thinking about the girls,' he said with that smug look that he has.

'What makes you think I fancied the girl at the barbecue?' He told me he could always tell when I fancied someone because I would stand there gawping at them with my mouth open. Well, if I'd turned on my charm, she wouldn't have been able to resist – after all, she was only human.

'Bollocks,' he said, 'you bottled it.'

'I didn't bottle it, I just felt a little bit embarrassed, that's all. I felt embarrassed because you were with me.'

'What's me being with you got to do with you being embarrassed? After all, she can't see me.'

'That's where you're wrong, she could see you because she asked me why my fingers were so fat and she asked me why I was limping when I walked. So I told her it was you that was making me limp, and it was you that was making my fingers fat, because you don't like me eating beef burgers and you don't like me drinking lager, because food and drink like that set your hormones off and make you grumpy.'

Uncle Arthur laughed at me and said, 'What did you say that for?' So I told him it was the first thing that came into my head. 'I didn't realise I embarrassed you so much,' he replied.

'Well you do now, so can we please just drop the subject?'

I know there are many people out there like myself who also suffer and struggle on a daily basis with this illness. Some people will have a far more aggressive form of Arthritis than mine, and there are some people that will have a less aggressive form, but we are all generally going through the same problems. Even though I know there are many people like myself, I still feel as though I am sometimes travelling alone with my illness. I feel I am travelling over land and seas on my own, and sometimes I feel god isn't looking over me. When I need his wind in my sails he sometimes isn't there. I do trust him, he just needs to breathe a little harder into my sails to keep me sailing along, that's all. When I ask myself what the future holds for me, three frightening words come rushing into my mind. The three words are: 'I don't know.'

I know my Uncle Arthur will grow grumpier and grumpier as the years pass by, so I know things will get worse for me. Like everybody else I have lots of ambitions, but because of my Uncle Arthur some of them are now beyond my reach. I have always dreamt of climbing Mount Everest, but can you imagine me telling Uncle Arthur I fancied climbing Everest? He would have a heart attack. But some of my ambitions are still possible so I must remain optimistic and chase those dreams, in fact I am going to chase those dreams, I have to.

That reminds me – it's Uncle Arthur's birthday next week, he probably thinks I am going to buy him his favourite stuff like drugs or a couple of bottles of cod liver oil, or some fresh fish. Well he can think again. I don't mind buying him the cod liver oil and maybe the fish, but there's no way he is getting any of those drugs, because like I say, when he has had them he pretends he has gone away, only to come back in a really bad mood, so he is simply not getting any of them. In fact, why should I buy him anything at all, because he won't appreciate it, he never does.

Anyway, I haven't forgiven him yet for the other day when we had a massive argument. He was bang out of order; he said he was sick of sleeping in just my body and threatened to move into the bodies of some of my family. I immediately thought of my ageing mother.

I have my good days and my bad days with Uncle Arthur, but because I am younger I can just about handle him. My mother is on her own, as my father passed away some time ago. She couldn't cope if Uncle Arthur decided to move in with her. I know she sometimes gets lonely and could do with some company, but not that sort of company. I know my mother would get really depressed if Uncle Arthur decided to move in with her. My mother likes to go dancing, it's really helped her cope with things and she has met some new friends, and so seems to be enjoying life a little bit more. She misses my father dearly, so she needs her dancing to help take her mind off things, if only for a while. If Uncle Arthur ever tried moving in with her and stopping her doing the things she likes, I would kick his head in.

Anyway, after our latest little dispute I had to find a way of stopping him moving into other people's bodies, especially my mother's. I have somehow got to stop him getting there. This is going to be a tough task because I can't just hire some hitman to take him out, that won't work because bullets can't kill him. No, I have got to box clever with this situation. If I can make as many people as possible aware of the disease – because that's what he is, Uncle Arthur is just a disease that won't go away – I will at least be making a start. I'm thinking the more people that learn about him and realise how horrible he is, and the suffering that he causes people for no apparent reason, then the hatred towards him will grow and grow. Now if he has any sense he will realise that there are thousands of people queuing up to kill him and he will leave town. Well, that's my thinking anyway, I don't know if it will work but it's worth a go.

It is a well-known fact that people like my Uncle Arthur don't like money. He knows that money can buy things that might kill him off. He knows that money can buy equipment and research, and he knows deep down that one day if enough money is raised he will be killed off. I know he doesn't want that, he would rather stay around and bring as much pain and misery into as many people's lives as possible. Well, I for one am not going to let that happen, so my quest is to tell the world about him.

Chapter Six

THE MARATHON

In fact I have already begun my quest, I started it last year. Me and Uncle Arthur had another argument. It started when I told him my intentions to tell the world about him. I told him I was going to tell as many people as I could what a really nasty piece of work he was. Well, he went mad because he doesn't like me being brave and standing up to him. He said that he had been around for years and not many people knew about him. I said, 'Well that's going to change, pal.'

He laughed and said, 'How do you intend to tell people and make them more aware of me? And more importantly, how are you going to make them listen to you?'

What he didn't know is that I had just won a place in the forthcoming London marathon. I had applied six months earlier but didn't say anything to him, as I had applied before but hadn't got in because they turn so many people down. Anyway, when I got the phone call to say I had got in I was overwhelmed and so excited. In six months' time I knew it was going to be me against Uncle Arthur in a running battle that would last for twenty-six point two miles. The reason I didn't tell Uncle Arthur I had got a place is because I know him only too well.

I knew he would try his best to stop me from training for it, and I knew that if I didn't train I had no chance of completing the marathon – therefore I would fail in my ultimate aim to beat my Uncle Arthur. It's just like being a boxer – if you don't train for the fight you will get beaten. So I had to train for the event behind Uncle Arthur's back. I had to train when he was sleeping, I had to train when he wasn't bugging me or hassling me. A good time to do this was when I had given him some of his favourite foods like fish and chicken and plenty of water. You see, things like fish and chicken are good for us both, especially when I was training for the marathon. I also knew I could fit some training in when he was enjoying some of his favourite warm weather, because as you know he doesn't bother me as much then. There were always going to be days when I couldn't train because he would know I was up to something, so I had to accept this and just be patient and train steadily and sensibly.

I really enjoyed the training because it was great trying to outmanoeuvre my Uncle Arthur. I really felt for the first time in ages that I was ready to take him on and show him I wasn't going to go down without a fight. So the night before the race I told him what I was going to do the next day. Well, he nearly choked. He said, 'What do you mean, you're going to do the London marathon?'

'You heard me,' I replied.

'Bollocks,' he said.

'Just watch me.'

'If you think I'm going to let you do the London marathon you must be dafter than I thought.'

'I don't care what you think. I'm going to do the marathon whether you like it or not.'

He started laughing at me and said, 'Even people who don't have to carry Arthritis round with them will struggle to complete the London marathon, so what chance have you got? Anyway, you haven't trained for it.'

'That's where you're wrong, clever clogs. I have been training, I've been training behind your back.'

'What do you mean?'

'I've been training when you've been asleep in the bit of warm weather we've had recently. And why do you think I've been filling you with all that chicken and fish and drowning you out with all that water?'

'I knew you were up to something,' he said. 'I wondered why you haven't been giving me as much of that lager as you normally do, and I was only thinking to myself the other day that you hadn't treated me to one of my favourite kebabs with all the trimmings on it for a while – and as for the fry-ups, well I've forgotten what they taste like.' At that point his face turned to anger and I could see he wasn't happy, so I thought it better to leave the room and go to bed for an early night; after all I didn't want to push my luck too far with him.

Anyway, I had managed to box clever and my training had gone well, and so came the big day. When I woke up in the morning I must admit I was quite nervous, as I hadn't challenged my Uncle Arthur to anything like this before.

The first thing I noticed that morning was that it was raining, and I realised that Uncle Arthur had probably ordered the bad weather himself as a way of denting my chances of finishing the race. Anyway, I kept telling myself that I had trained well and was going to beat him, I had to beat him because I also had a lot of money riding on it. After nagging everybody half to death to sponsor me in my quest, I soon had every Tom, Dick and Harry on my sponsorship form, which was great because the more people on my form the more people were getting to know about Arthritis, which after all is my aim. I didn't mind that Uncle Arthur had ordered the rain and wind because I had one last trick up my sleeve. Just before the race I was going to cover my body in a muscle-warming substance.

It is something footballers use in the winter. I knew that covering my body in this substance would give me at least a couple of hours head start on Uncle Arthur. You see, he hates me wearing stuff like that because he knows it warms my body up, and if my body is warm he can't trouble me in the way he would like to. I'd like to wear this stuff more often but I can't because it stinks. I would hate to have people look at me and say to their friends, 'I don't like the smell of that bloke's after-shave.'

When I got to the start line I was really excited. There was a great atmosphere as there were thousands of other people running. They all had their own reasons for running and I had mine. To tell people why I was running I decided to wear a vest, which basically said I am running to kill Arthritis. At first I was going to wear a vest saying, I am running to kill my Uncle Arthur, but I didn't want people constantly asking me what it meant so I decided to use his common name.

When the race started I felt good, and even though it was raining and cold, I said, 'Right, Uncle Arthur, for the next twenty-six point two miles it's just you and me.' He said I had cheated by covering my body with the muscle-warming substance. I said, 'No I haven't, that's quite within the rules.'

The next thing he said to me worried me a little bit.

'Enjoy the first half of the race and enjoy the crowds clapping you around, because in the second part I am going to give you hell.'

Anyway, I did enjoy the first part of the race and it was great to have the huge crowd clapping and cheering me on, but at approximately fifteen miles into the race

Uncle Arthur hit me with everything he had. I was in trouble. He kept saying to me I wasn't going to finish the race and he was going to grind me into the ground mile by mile. He wasn't kidding, he really started to attack my feet. He knew that if he caused enough damage to my feet I wouldn't be able to finish the race. They started to swell up mile by mile and the pain at twenty miles was almost too much.

I stopped to gather my thoughts. Should I give in now and be proud that I had managed to complete twenty miles, or should I be stubborn and try to reach the finish? Well, it helps to be stubborn sometimes and so I plodded on.

At this stage in the race I was near the back of the field, but the main thing is I was still in the field and I had to keep thinking tactics against my Uncle Arthur. At that point I loosened the laces on my trainers, this would give Uncle Arthur a bit more room to move in and give me a bit more of a chance of finishing. But this only helped a little and at twenty-three miles he was attacking the whole of my body as he was determined I wouldn't finish the race.

I felt cold, wet and demoralised. He was not only attacking my body, he was also attacking my mind.

I felt nauseated and had lost all sense of time.

Even though I was surrounded by some of the most famous landmarks in the world, I just didn't seem to notice them.

But I kept going and at twenty-four miles something a little strange happened. An old man passed me, I am guessing he was about seventy years old. As he passed me he realised I was really struggling, I was barely able to walk. He stopped and said 'Come on son, you can do it – only two more miles to go.' He looked at my vest and said 'Arthritis?'

I said yes, and looked at his vest, which said 'Multiple Sclerosis'. I said, 'That's a good cause you're running for.'

He said, 'Yes, and so is yours.' Then the defining moment came – I asked him how much money he had managed to raise. He put his arm around me and said, 'I will have raised nothing if I don't get you to the finishing line.'

It was like he was going to battle Uncle Arthur with me for the remaining two miles. His own determination to finish gave me that one last bit of steam I needed, and so we set off together. During those difficult last two miles we chatted a little. He told me his son had Multiple Sclerosis and that's why the charity was so close to his heart. He asked me why I was running for Arthritis. 'I suffer from the condition,' I replied. He said I was brave to be tackling the London marathon with that condition. 'I'm not brave,' I replied, 'I'm fortunate.' My thoughts for a moment turned to his son. I said I was fortunate to be able to run and raise awareness of the problem, and I felt even more fortunate and proud to be running with the likes of this man. At that point I told him to run on ahead of me, I told him I didn't want to hold him up any longer.

He said, 'Promise me you will finish.'

'I promise,' I said and thanked him for his words of encouragement and understanding, and then off he went.

I started to jog again myself as I could see the twenty-five mile marker approaching and I could see Buckingham Palace. At that point Uncle Arthur reminded me he was not going to go down without a fight and pounded my body again with his anger. But it was too late for him because at that point I knew I was going to finish, and just to really upset him, when I came level with Buckingham Palace I said to him, 'Why don't you go and have a cup of tea with the Queen?' It's quite strange because I enjoyed that last mile more than any of the others. Even though I was dead on my feet it was a great feeling knowing I was going to finish. I could see the finishing line in the distance and the crowds were all clapping and cheering, just as they had clapped and cheered me and the other runners all the way around the course.

The moment I finally crossed the line was one I will never forget. I had so many emotions running through me, a mixture of elation and excitement and happiness and relief. I remember it was still raining but amidst the rain on my face there was a little tear that had rolled down my cheek, one little tear of happiness. And so for that one day I had conquered Uncle Arthur. I knew deep down it would be a rare victory against him but that one day will live with me forever.

I would like to say to the people who have Arthritis, let's not walk in silence with the problem, let's tell people about it because the more people we tell the fewer people will be affected by it in the future.

Chapter Seven

SYMPTOMS

If people can avoid Arthritis, then they must try their best to do so, because the illness is very clever. It doesn't warn you when it is coming, it just creeps up on you – so batten down the hatches now. I remember when it crept up on me.

I remember a dull aching pain in my hand. At first I thought I had just sprained it or something and that the pain would just disappear, but I was wrong. The pain continued and gradually started to get worse. I decided to go and see my doctor just to get it checked out: it proved to be a bad day for me. The doctor examined me and told me I had Arthritis. At first I didn't understand. I thought Arthritis just affected older people, and so I said, 'Are you sure?'

He said, 'Yes, you have Arthritis.'

'You're joking,' I said. 'I'm only twenty-seven years old.'

The doctor said, 'Yes, you have been dealt a rather bad card being so young.'

And so there started my battle with Uncle Arthur. People who have Arthritis have one person to convince before anybody else that they can beat or at least try and cope with the illness and live their lives the best they can, and that person is themselves. I have found out that this is easier said than done, but it is vital that we try.

One of the most important factors in the fight against this illness is exercise. It is vital that we try and keep ourselves mobile, and a good way to do this is to find some form of exercise that suits the individual sufferer.

I wouldn't recommend to any Arthritis sufferer that they should try and complete the marathon, because that would be bad advice. I have always wanted to do the marathon, and when the chance came along I just couldn't resist. Completing it was a triumph for me in my personal battle with this illness, and it was a day I will never forget, but I know deep down that the pounding my body took, not just on the day but also from all the training I did leading up to it, will not have done me any good in the long term. So it is extremely important to exercise without causing damage to the joints. I decided to take on the marathon because I wanted to raise money and therefore awareness of the problem, and I felt young and fit enough to do it. That was my decision alone. If an Arthritis sufferer is going to attempt the marathon or anything else that is demanding and stressful, it will be their own decision to do so, and that decision should be respected.

The way I like to keep myself fit in general is to take a steady walk of a mile or so maybe twice a week. Another thing I like to do is to go swimming, because as everybody knows swimming is very good for you, especially for someone that suffers from Arthritis, because we are not applying any direct pressure to the joints. This is probably our best option in the quest to stay mobile and fit.

I suppose it's easy to say that exercise is crucial for the Arthritis sufferer, but I do know that there are a lot of people, old and young, that simply can't manage any exercise at all due to the illness, and for these people it is crucial that a cure is found sooner rather than later.

Chapter Eight

CHILDREN AND THE ELDERLY

Today I read something that made me feel very sad indeed. It was an article in my local paper about an eleven-year-old boy who suffers from a rare form of Arthritis called Juvenile Idiopathic Arthritis. He finds it difficult to wash, dress and feed himself on a daily basis, and he has to take antibiotics to fend off infections. He can also no longer take part in sporting events at school which involve contact, and he has to stay inside during dinner and lunch breaks because of the risk of getting injured.

When I read this lad's story it made me realise once again something which deep down I already knew: there is always somebody worse off than ourselves. No matter how bad we sometimes feel about our own problems there is always someone worse off. In the article it states how the young lad is trying his best not to let his illness get him down, which is bravery in itself. I am inspired by this young man because he and his mother are organising a charity walk in the near future in the hope of raising money and awareness of Arthritis in children, which is a great idea.

So there is only one thing for it, I will need to get my training shoes out again and join him – and hopefully many others – on the charity walk. I wish him all the best for the future.

Arthritis is in itself a sad, lonely and painful illness, and should be taken very seriously. As I have stated earlier, it stops you from carrying out the most basic functions in life that most people take for granted. Think of this: I am only thirty-six years old and yet I really struggle on a daily basis to carry out very simple functions without being in pain.

As I battle on with my illness there never seems to be a day goes by when I don't think about the elderly people that have this same terrible problem. I hate to think of them living on their own, having nobody at their side to talk to because this is a lonely disease as it is. Whenever I am struggling with my Arthritis and feeling sorry for myself, I just stop and think to myself, hang on a minute, if I am struggling at my age with this problem, what must it be like for the elderly? How are they coping?

My heart bleeds for these people and I so often wonder to myself how they cope. Because of my age there are still many things I can do in my quest to lead as normal a life as possible, which I suppose makes me fortunate compared to some of the elderly people who simply can't manage any more. Many of these elderly people will have lived through the war and will have fought for their country as fit young men and women, and so to be brought down by this terrible illness is a total injustice to them.

Chapter Nine

THE FRIENDLY CHAT WITH UNCLE ARTHUR

I decided I needed to sit down with Uncle Arthur and have a chat with him, a civilised chat where we wouldn't end up arguing as usual.

Last night I seized my chance. He was sitting watching TV, it was early evening and we had just had tea. I had purposely eaten a healthy meal to get him in a good mood. Anyway, I sat down beside him and said, 'Uncle Arthur, can we have a chat?'

'What about?' he said

'You and me,' I replied.

'What's the point in us chatting? We always fall out and the reason we fall out is because you don't like me living in your body, and because you don't want me living in your body it makes me feel unwelcome.'

'That's what I want to talk to you about,' I said. 'If we're going to live together we need to come to some sort of compromise.'

'What do you mean?' he replied.

'Well we need to find some sort of middle ground where I can enjoy my life a little bit better than I do at the moment, and where you can have a bit more room to sleep in without affecting me.'

'How are we going to do that?' he replied.

So I said to him, 'Even though you're my Uncle Arthur I don't really know too much about you. I don't know the fundamental things about you.'

'Like what?' he said.

'I need to know more about these secrets you've been keeping to yourself for all these years. How have you managed to keep medical science away from you for so long? Why in this day and age do people still not know the ways in which you like to operate? Like for example, why do you like to attack when it's damp and cold? And why are you less aggressive when it's warm weather? And why do certain foods we eat set you off? And I've always wondered why you like to attack the joints?'

'That's my little secret,' he said.

'I know it's your little secret, but that's why I've asked you to sit down for a chat with me.'

'Why should I tell you my secrets?' he replied.

'Because I want to live a better life for myself. I'm

sick of being in pain all the time and I'm sick of not being able to do some of the things that people take for granted on a daily basis.'

A sad look came upon my face and Uncle Arthur spotted this. 'Carry on,' he said.

'Well, I miss things like a nice game of golf with my mates because you won't let me grip the clubs without giving me all this pain and discomfort, and I hate sitting at home on my own knowing that all my mates are out playing golf and enjoying themselves.'

At this point a guilty look comes on his face; maybe I am getting through to him at last? So I continue to tell him about the other things I miss, like going to the gym and being able to grip the handles on the machines like the rowing machine. I used to like going on the rowing machine because it was a good way of keeping fit. If I went on it now I would probably sink. Uncle Arthur chuckles to himself at my little joke. I think it's the first time I have seen him laugh and with that a thought crosses my mind. I wonder if he never laughs because he is sad and lonely as I sometimes am.

'What else do you miss? he said.

We had now talked for half an hour without arguing and that's a record for us. I said, 'I miss the simple things, like being able to walk without limping and being able to do simple things with my hands.'

'Name me a couple,' he said.

'Well, for a start I can only fill the kettle half full

because I can't pick it up properly when it's full because the sudden pain makes me tilt the kettle and risk spilling hot water over myself. And one thing I would really like is to be able to grip my hairbrush properly, this would give myself a better chance of having a better-looking hairstyle.'

'That's just an excuse,' he said. 'You'll always have a crap hairstyle.'

'Cheeky sod,' I replied with a smile.

'Are you saying I'm so bad you can't even use your hairbrush properly?'

'It's true, I can't.'

He paused for a moment, then under his breath I heard him mumble the word shit, as if he was realising he didn't know he was that bad. 'Anything else?' he said.

'Yes, will you please let me out of the house in the morning when we've had frost the night before?'

'I don't understand,' he said. So I told him that when we have had frost the night before, the door frames swell up and jam because they are made of wood, and because they jam I can't grip the handle hard enough to open the door, and because of this I have to ring work and go through the embarrassment of having to explain to my boss that I am going to be late because I can't undo the doors.

Again he laughs, but this time in disbelief. I think he is slowly realising what an absolute swine he is. 'Is there anything else you'd like to get off your chest?' he said.

'Oh yes, there is one other thing,' I said to him.

'What's that?' he replied.

'Well, as you know, I like to play the piano because it relaxes me when I've had a bad day at work or when I'm just generally stressed out with things. But because you decide to make my hands and fingers swell up it stops me from playing because I can't adjust my fingers to the keys without being in pain, and if I'm in pain I can't concentrate on what I'm doing.

He then replied with some more of his dry sense of humour, 'Have you ever considered that the reason I stop you from playing is because you are affecting my ears with the way in which you play it?' At this point I sensed he was joking with me, because I am not a bad pianist – okay I am never going to be Jools Holland but I am not that bad. At this stage me and Uncle Arthur seemed to be quite relaxed with each other and this is a rarity. His next question caught me by surprise.

'Why do you swear a lot?' he asked me. I thought for a moment and then told him it was the frustration and pain and sadness of having to carry him round with me on a daily basis which leads me to swear a lot. 'Oh,' he said with a sad look on his face. I then apologised for swearing at him and calling him a bastard. 'Apology accepted,' he replied. He then apologised to me for calling me an idiot.

'Apology accepted,' I replied.

There was another slight pause then Uncle Arthur calmly said, 'If I'm going to give you a better lifestyle, you need to help me.'

'What do you mean?' I replied.

'You need to help me by first helping yourself. If you want me to be less aggressive with you then you need to start looking after your body, which I live in. Once you start to do that more often, the easier it will be for you to understand some of the mysterious ways in which I work.' He went on to tell me that I know the sort of foods which set him off.

'Yes I know,' I replied.

'Then think about it,' he said.

I knew what he was saying but I sort of like my diet. As I was thinking about what he had told me, he said to me, 'The key to the secret is moderation. If you want to drink lager or eat kebabs then do so in moderation and not every night, which is what you do at the moment.'

I knew he was right, and maybe for a change I should listen to him. I need to help myself in order to help him. I then referred back to some of the earlier questions that I had asked him, like why is he less aggressive when it's warm weather? And why does he get so angry when it is cold and damp? When I ask him to explain these things he says he can't.

'Why not?' I replied. He said he didn't know, he doesn't really understand himself why he operates in the way he does. He told me it's the demons in his head which set him off and he has no way of controlling them. He also went on to say that he doesn't just attack humans – he attacks animals as well. This I didn't realise and it made me pause for a moment, At least I can tell people when I am in pain but the animals can't, which concerns me. At this point I looked at my swollen fingers and felt that there is a common sadness between me and my Uncle Arthur, and I now think I know what it is. I don't really want him here, but I also think he doesn't really want to be here himself.

For the next five minutes we sat and stared at each other. I stared down at him through my hands and feet and he stared back at me: he is the swelling. At that point I decided to thank him for our little chat and suggest an early night. He agreed.

In the morning when I woke up I didn't really feel in any great pain, maybe Uncle Arthur had enjoyed our little chat the night before? 'Morning,' I said to him.

'Morning,' he replied.

'What do you fancy for breakfast?' I asked him.

'Whatever you're having I'll have too,' he replied.

'Would you mind if I have a big fry-up?'

'If you want a big greasy fry-up I'll allow you to have one without causing you any grief.' Great, I thought to myself. 'Don't get used to it,' he said, 'it's only a one-off.'

'I won't,' I replied.

So as we sat down to a really nice fry-up, he said to me, 'Do you remember what I told you last night?'

'Yes, you said eat and drink the things you like but only in moderation.'

'Correct,' he said.

If only I could find the incentive to do that, I thought to myself. He seemed to know what I was thinking and said to me, 'Let me give you the incentive. If you eat and drink sensibly for the next week I will give you a day off from me for showing some will-power.'

'Do you mean it?' I replied.

'Yes,' he said. 'I'll give you the full day to yourself so you can enjoy some of the things you've been wishing for.'

'You're on,' I said.

And so for the next week I eat and drink sensibly. I take on as much water as possible even though it is making me piss like a circus horse. I eat plenty of fresh fish and chicken and try to stuff as many vegetables down my neck as possible. At the end of the week I ask my Uncle Arthur whether I have completed the task.

'Yes,' he replied. 'It's amazing what you can achieve with a little bit of will-power. Right,' he said, 'which day would you like me to leave you alone?'

I thought for a moment and then realised that the coming Friday was a friend's birthday and that he was having a party, so I told Uncle Arthur, 'I'll have this Friday off, please.'

'Okay, no problem. But remember – the deal is for one day only and it will end at midnight on Friday.'

Bloody hell, I suddenly feel like Cinderella. 'Okay,' I told him, 'twenty-four hours it is.' And so I look forward to Friday.

Chapter Ten

THE DREAM DAY UNCLE ARTHUR GRANTS ME

When Friday arrived I was really excited. A full day without Uncle Arthur ... this was something I had dreamed of for the last few years. Anyway, without further ado let me tell you what I did.

On waking up in the morning free from pain I decided to sneak another one of those lovely greasy fry-ups, washed down with a couple of mugs of coffee – remember, you should always try to start your day with a good solid meal, no matter what you suffer from.

As I am sitting eating my breakfast I look out of the window, and it looks lovely and sunny. I am getting a sudden urge to go for a little jog – once the breakfast has settled of course. It will be the first time I have run since the marathon.

So after my breakfast had settled I got my running shoes on, and off I went. I decided to take the same route I took when I was in the early stages of my training for the marathon, only this time I was not in any pain or discomfort, which was nice. I didn't want to push myself too far so I decided to just do a steady couple of miles, just to blow the cobwebs out of my system. I really enjoyed the run and when I got back I took a nice cold shower followed by some lunch, which was a couple of pies from the local pie shop. Apart from looking forward to tonight's party, I also knew I had the afternoon to fill. There was only one thing I wanted to do: yes, you guessed it, a game of golf. So I got on the phone and rounded up a couple of my mates, as I knew they had taken the day off in preparation for the party.

When we arrived at the golf club I remember walking down to the first tee: it was a really nice feeling, especially as it was my first game for nearly three years. I am not going to talk you through the whole round, but I would like you to know it was the best feeling I had felt for ages.

I knew I had missed playing golf, but I didn't realise how much until I was actually out there playing. I was really relaxed and didn't half enjoy the sight of the beautiful course we were playing on. The peacefulness of it all was wonderful. I must admit, though, I didn't really play that well, but that was understandable as I was almost as rusty as my clubs. I ended up finishing with the worst score out of the four of us that were playing, but that didn't matter as I was buzzing. We then finished the round off with a couple of pints in the clubhouse, as you do. I really enjoyed my afternoon, and to make it even better I wasn't in any pain. Uncle Arthur had so far kept his word.

As I was getting ready for the party a thought crossed my mind. I wondered what Uncle Arthur was doing with himself? Don't get me wrong: I wasn't missing him; I was just wondering what he might be doing.

I guess he was probably out somewhere with his best mate Stress. I can just imagine the conversation between those two. Arthur would probably say to Stress, 'What have you been up to today?' And Stress would reply, 'Oh, I've just spoiled a few more people's day just by walking round with them.'

'Me too,' Uncle Arthur would reply. 'I've stopped a few people from doing normal day-to-day things they enjoy doing just by causing them some pain.'

Then they would probably raise their glasses and say here's to causing people grief and pain.

Anyway, never mind those two. I am getting ready for the party, and as I stand in front of the mirror it's nice to be able to hold my hairbrush properly. As I am brushing my hair a thought comes into my mind: Uncle Arthur was right, I have got a crap hairstyle.

And so the big night arrives and as I walk into the party it's a nice feeling knowing I can have a few drinks without having to worry about the consequences, and I can go around shaking people's hands without Uncle Arthur thinking someone is trying to throttle him.

The night is going well, I am on my fifth pint and have already hit the dance floor a couple of times. I am not the best of dancers but after a couple of beers you think you are John Travolta. As I stand at the bar I notice a girl sitting at a table on the other side of the dance floor. She is beautiful and what's more she seems to be looking straight at me.

At this point a couple of thoughts go dashing through my mind: is the beer taking over, is she really looking at me or is she looking at somebody else nearby? The only people I am standing with are a couple of my mates and they are as ugly as sin, so she must be looking at me. So I test the water and throw her a little smile. She smiles back. Oh my God, she is looking at me.

Now, I have never been the best at going over to girls and starting a conversation, because I have always been a bit shy, but I knew deep down I had to get over my reservations and make a move. I suddenly started to think about the girl at the barbecue: would she start asking questions about my fat fingers and would I be embarrassed at telling her I had Arthritis? Then I remembered that Uncle Arthur had given me the night off, and this was my big chance. I took a big gulp of my pint and started to walk across the dance floor towards her.

When I arrived at her table, I saw that she was the most beautiful girl I had ever seen. She said hello and I seemed lost for words. I felt like just asking her for a light and walking back to the bar, but then I thought to myself, don't be daft, you don't smoke. So I plucked up the courage and asked her to dance. To my astonishment she said 'yes'. I said, 'Are you sure?'

She got up, grabbed me by the arm and dragged me onto the dance floor. That must be a yes, then.

I remember the song that was playing: it was 'Come on Eileen' by Dexy's Midnight Runners, one of my favourites. As we boogied away, I knew the girl was a little tipsy herself as she kept standing on my feet, but I didn't care. I was in love.

I am like that – I fall in love quicker than anybody else in the world. I have always been the same, maybe I just think I am in love when really I am not, I don't know. Anyway, after dancing for a while we went and sat down at the bar for a drink. I remember my mates looking over and shouting out the usual remarks – watch him love, you don't know where he's been. So I told her to just ignore them, as they were just a bunch of drunkards. One of them shouted out, 'What time does your wife want you home?'

Shit, I thought, it's not the wife I need to worry about, it's Uncle Arthur – he's going to come back into my body at twelve o'clock. The girl noticed my concerned look and said, 'Have you got a wife?'

'No,' I replied, 'I've got something worse.'

'What's that?' she said.

'Oh, nothing,' I said, 'it doesn't really matter.'

'Come on,' she said, 'I want to know.'

I thought to myself, I must tell her about the Arthritis because if I don't I'll be really annoyed with myself for letting embarrassment get the better of me, just as it did at the barbecue. I also realised that if I was still sitting with her at twelve o'clock Uncle Arthur would come back into my fingers and swell them up, and she would notice.

So I took a deep breath and said, 'I have Arthritis.'

She looked a little puzzled and said, 'Oh.'

'I've had it for nine years,' I told her.

'Aren't you a little young to have arthritis?' she replied.

'Yes, I've just been dealt a bad card, that's all.'

What she said next really cheered me up. In fact it made my night.

'Just because you have Arthritis it doesn't mean I don't like you the same.'

'Doesn't it put you off me?' I asked.

'Why should it?' she said.

She was right: why should somebody be put of somebody else just because they have Arthritis? As we chatted away about my condition we talked a lot about the people that were worse off than ourselves and agreed that we shouldn't always complain about our own problems. We talked about the people starving in Africa and the homeless people that have to live on the streets, and the poor children that have no parents and have nobody to love them. These people are but a few that we talked about, and one day it would be nice to try and help these people in some way. As my lovely new companion and I talked, I noticed the time on my watch, it was quarter past twelve. I looked at my fingers: they weren't swollen. Uncle Arthur hadn't arrived back yet. Maybe he was pissed up somewhere with his mate Stress, or maybe they had just got lucky with the girls themselves?

As the night drew to a close, the girl and I had a little smooch on the dance floor. We danced the last dance, a perfect end to a perfect day. Afterwards we arranged to meet up to see each other again.

I'd had a brilliant night and a brilliant day without having to worry about my Uncle Arthur.

The morning after, I was sitting in the kitchen having a cup of tea, thinking about the brilliant day I had yesterday, but more importantly I was thinking about the lovely girl I had met. Just then Uncle Arthur walked in. 'Morning,' I said to him. 'Morning,' he replied, and asked how my day had been.

'Absolutely fantastic,' I told him. 'How was yours?'

'Not bad,' he said, so I asked him what he did. He said he went out with his mate Stress.

'Thought so,' I said.

'How did you know I was out with Stress?'

'Because you two go hand in hand.'

'Yes, I suppose we do,' he replied. He then asked me how my day had been without him. I paused and told him calmly that it had been one of the best days of my life. 'Don't tell me you fell in love again?' he said. I thought of the girl and smiled. 'I knew it,' he said, 'I just knew it, the minute I let you out of my sight you go and fall in love again.'

'Uncle Arthur, I haven't fallen in love, I've just met somebody really nice, that's all.'

'I knew as soon as I walked into the kitchen you'd met someone.'

'How did you work that one out?'

'Because normally when you've been out the night before and haven't met anybody you spend the next day walking round with a face that could sink a thousand ships. But now you're sat there looking like the cat that got the cream.'

'I just feel happy today, that's all.'

'It's about time you had some luck with the girls.'

'What do you mean by that?'

He said, 'Let's face it, you normally don't have much luck with the girls. You always seem to crash and burn like you did with that girl at the barbecue.'

'I didn't crash and burn with that girl at the barbecue. I never even managed to take off in the first place.'

He then just smiled and asked if the girl had a name.

'Yes, Uncle Arthur, her name is Annabel.'

'Annabel. That's a nice name,' he replied.

'Yes, it is, and she was beautiful to match.'

He then got a little excited and asked if he could be the best man.

'Hang on a minute, Uncle Arthur – I've only just met the girl!'

'Tell me more about her,' he said.

'Like I say, I only met her last night, so I didn't really get to know that much about her.'

He paused while he thought about his next question, then looked me in the eye and asked, 'Was it love at first sight?' I tried to brush his question aside and asked him kindly to stop quizzing me, but he was insistent. 'Was it love at first sight? He asked again.

I looked him in the eyes and smiled, and simply said, 'Yes, it was love at first sight.'

He jumped to his feet and before I could get another word in he started to sing: 'He's getting married in the morning, ding dong the bells are going to chime, pull out the stopper, let's have a whopper, but get him to the church on time.'

'Uncle Arthur, will you please stop embarrassing me!'

He then put his arm around me and said, 'I am not trying to embarrass you, I am just happy for you, that's all.'

'Uncle Arthur, I want you to calm down and listen to me good. You granted me yesterday without you, which

I made the most of: I had a fantastic day being able to do the normal day to day things which I miss, and to round it off I met a lovely girl by the name of Annabel, who brought a moment of happiness into my life, and that's all there is to it.'

He paused and said, 'Well, are you going to see Annabel again?'

'Yes Uncle Arthur, I am going to see her again,' I replied.

'Good, well let's hope it takes your mind off me for a while.' Yes, let's hope it does, I thought to myself. He then came and sat at the table with me and said, 'Would you like to have more of those days?'

'Of course I would,' I replied.

'Well, if you listen to the things I've told you about watching what you eat and watching how you control your lifestyle, then you'll have a chance to lead a better life for yourself.'

He then brought me back down to earth and told me that the day I had enjoyed yesterday was just a one-off and would always be a one-off until society found a cure for him. I knew he was right, and accepted that I would have to continue to take my good days without him along with the bad days I would have with him.

Chapter Eleven

BIRTHDAYS, CHRISTMAS AND ANNIVERSARIES

Over the weeks that followed, me and Uncle Arthur would share another of my birthdays and another Christmas together. I have never really been that big on celebrating birthdays. I don't know why, maybe it's because I am now clocking on a bit. On the morning of my birthday I woke up, as you do (well at least you hope you do) and Uncle Arthur was there as usual.

'Good morning and happy birthday,' he said. As I lifted my head off the pillow and sat on the edge of the bed, he once again wished me happy birthday.

'What's good about it?' I snapped.

'Bloody hell, you are in a bad mood this morning,' he replied.

'No, I'm not in a bad mood, I'm just not that thrilled at turning thirty-seven years old, that's all.'

'What's wrong with thirty-seven?' he asked.

'What's wrong with it? I'll tell you what is wrong with it – the fact that I've just turned thirty-seven means I'm nearly forty. That's what's wrong with it.'

'What's wrong with being forty? I'm hundreds of years old, and you're moaning about being on your way to forty?'

He was starting to get on my nerves. So I said to him, 'Being on my way to forty doesn't exactly give me the urge to do back-flips off the wardrobe, does it?'

Well, he just looked at me as though I was a bit daft, and then he came out with another one of his little reality speeches. 'You should celebrate every birthday, because you never know – it could be your last. And you should also be thankful you have some of your health left.'

At that point I interrupted him. 'If you would piss off, I'd have all of my health left.'

'Yes, well I can't do that, so you'll just have to put up with me, at least until some smartarse finds a cure for me.'

'Yes, well, if the person that does find a cure for you comes riding along on his great white horse I shall be the first to shake his hand.'

Uncle Arthur gave me another daft look and realised that I was not in a very good mood, so he told me he was nipping out for a paper and to get some fresh air. 'Good idea,' I said, 'and don't bother rushing back.'

Because Arthritis is at its worst in the mornings, it can spoil some of your big days before they have even started.

Imagine waking up on, say, your wedding day in pain: it wouldn't be very nice, would it? After all the planning and organisation you have put into the big day, Arthritis would still try and spoil it for you. Or can you imagine planning to ask someone to marry you, and when the big day finally arrives you get down on bended knee, ask the person to marry you, and hopefully they say yes, but then you can't get back up because of the Arthritis. Now that would be rather embarrassing, but the Arthritis wouldn't care, because he just doesn't mind spoiling somebody's big day or big moment.

Anyway, my thirty-seventh birthday gradually got better for me as the day went on. I ended up going out with a few friends. Being my friends, they wouldn't let me pay for a single drink all night, and because of that I felt really appreciated, which is always nice, and because of that it made for quite a nice birthday. One of the key secrets in keeping my Uncle Arthur quiet is having something to take your mind off it, so being in good company and having a good laugh is a good way of doing it.

And so my birthday slowly lapsed away and I was now heading towards thirty-eight. There would, however, be another occasion to mark before that birthday – in fact it would be an occasion to mark even before Christmas this year.

It was a morning early in December, and as I woke up I could hear some noise downstairs, and couldn't really understand what it was. I went down to check it out. When I opened the kitchen door, to my relief it was Uncle Arthur making breakfast. 'What are you doing?' I asked him.

'What's it look like? I'm making us breakfast, in fact I'm making us one of your favourite greasy fry-ups.'

'Why are you doing that? I normally do all the cooking.'

'Yes, well today I'm in a good mood so I'm doing the cooking, and if you don't mind I'd like you to go and sit down at the table. It'll be ready in a couple of minutes.'

'I don't understand, Uncle Arthur, why do you suddenly think you're Gordon Ramsay?'

'I don't think I'm Gordon Ramsay, I'm just in a good mood, that's all. Anyway, I wouldn't be Gordon Ramsay, I'd be Delia Smith. She's got a bit more class than him.'

'Yes, well it doesn't really matter to me which chef you'd rather be, I just want to know why you've woken me up this early to cook me breakfast?'

'I'm sorry to wake you, I was going to bring you breakfast in bed,' he said.

A puzzled look arrived upon my face and Uncle

Arthur spotted this. He turned the pans off and said to me, 'You've forgotten, haven't you?'

'Forgotten what?'

'It's our anniversary today,' he told me.

'Our anniversary? I don't understand.'

He then started to laugh out loud. 'It's ten years since we met, it's ten years since that first doctor told you the bad news that you had me.'

I started to think back. He was right, it was ten years to the day since I was first diagnosed with Arthritis. I started to stare into space as I thought back over those ten years and started to recall all the ups and downs with him, from the times I had coped quite well with him to the times that I hadn't, and to the times that I had laughed with him, to the times that I had cried with him. Even though it was our tenth anniversary together it wasn't a day of celebration, so I told him: 'Having you with me for the past ten years is certainly no excuse for me to be happy and celebrate.'

'Suit yourself,' he said. 'Don't celebrate with me. I'll just eat my breakfast on my own, and if you're not going to eat yours I'll eat it for you.'

'You can have it. I've suddenly lost my appetite.'

Whilst he was eating his breakfast I said to him, 'Uncle Arthur, do you remember the other morning when you were feeling down in the dumps?'

'Which other morning?' he replied.

'The other morning when you were ranting and

raving about people all over the world hating you for bringing pain and misery into their lives.'

'What about it?' he said with a sheepish look on his face.

'Don't you think you're being a little bit two-faced?'

'What do you mean, two-faced?' he said with a mouthful of sausage.

After reminding him of his table manners, I told him that even though he was down in the dumps because he realised that people all over the world hated him, he still had the face to celebrate being with someone for ten years. He then put his knife and fork down, took a gulp from his teacup and said to me that he was only celebrating his remaining existence and that ten years with someone is a milestone. He then went on to remind me of why I should celebrate every birthday. 'Existence,' he said, 'that's why I'm celebrating ten years with you, just as you should celebrate your continuing existence when you reach each of your birthdays, even if you do think you're getting old.'

I suppose his words did sort of make sense, but I was not going to admit it to him, because that would give him the upper hand again. He finished his breakfast, got up and then ran upstairs, singing to himself.

For the next few days I didn't really see too much of Uncle Arthur. I don't know why, but he never seems to trouble me that much when we are approaching

Christmas. I really enjoy the build-up to Christmas: there is just something about it that makes me feel really good. I love walking through the town centre on a cold dark night when all the Christmas lights are on and all the usual Christmas songs are being played while I am trying to complete my Christmas shopping, which in itself is a task, especially for a bloke. It is probably my biggest task of the year, trying to find something for everyone that they will like. Maybe the reason Uncle Arthur goes absent without leave during this time is because I have something to take my mind off him, like completing my Christmas shopping for my ever-growing family.

I didn't see Uncle Arthur again until two days later when he woke me up early one morning. He was jumping about by the window saying, 'Come and look! Quick, come and look!'

'Look at what?' I replied.

'It's snowing! The snow has come down and everything is white,' he said with excitement in his voice.

'Well, it will be white if it's been snowing won't it?' He gave me a sharp look and told me to stop being sarcastic.

'I'm going back to bed, it's too early to be getting up just because it's been snowing.'

Then he came and jumped on the bed at the side of me, and asked if we could go for a snowball fight. 'No, Uncle Arthur, we can't go for a snowball fight.'

'Why not?' he asked.

'You know why not, you know I can't make snowballs while you're in my hands.'

He then thought for a moment and said, 'Well, what about if I left your hands, would you have a snowball fight with me then?'

'You know it's hard for you to leave my hands when it's cold, because cold is your favourite weather, so how do you intend leaving my hands while we have a snowball fight?'

'There is a way,' he said.

'What's that?' I replied suspiciously.

'You can give me something you haven't given me for a long time.'

'What's that?' I said even more suspiciously.

He paused and said calmly, 'You can give me some of those drugs.'

'No way. You're not getting any of them, you know what you're like when you wake up after taking things like that, you're like a bear with a sore head.'

'Oh please give me some, please give me some, I've forgotten what they taste like it's been that long.'

'Why should I give you some? I know what you'll do, you'll take the tablets and then calm down for a while, but when the effects of the tablets wear off you'll be in an angry mood and cause me even more pain. So why should I give you some?'

'Because I want to have a snowball fight with you, and because it's Christmas.'

He was right, it was Christmas. Maybe I should give him some for a treat? I looked out of the window myself, and it was beautiful, just a pure blanket of snow. I then began to remember playing in the snow as a kid and having snowball fights and lots of fun. I had to give myself the best chance of enjoying this Christmas and everything that came with it, so I told Uncle Arthur he could have some of the drugs – but only this once. He jumped up and down with delight and thanked me for my kind gesture.

When he eventually calmed down he told me he knew why I couldn't always give him the tablets to keep him at bay. He said, 'I know you're trying not to rely on the tablets, and that is right because you're still at a young age.'

His last words on this subject of tablets will probably always stay with me. He simply said, 'Only take the tablets when you really have to.'

'Okay,' I said, 'I'll try my best to do that. Now, are we going for this snowball fight or what?'

Later that evening me and Uncle Arthur were feeling a little bit exhausted after our snowball fight, so we both put our feet up ready for a good old-fashioned pipe-and-slippers night. Uncle Arthur asked if I had enjoyed the snowball fight. Yes, I had, it had been good fun and sort of took me back to my childhood. 'Did you enjoy it?' I asked him back.

'Yes,' he replied, and said especially as he had got the best shot in.

'No you didn't get the best shot in. I did.'

Then he laughed out loud and said to me, 'That shot that hit you right between the eyes must be affecting your memory.'

'Oh yes, that shot. Okay, I agree it was a good shot but I still say it was a lucky one.'

A few seconds later I heard him mutter something under his breath. 'Did you say something?' I asked him.

'Yes,' he said, 'I asked if you had bought me a present for Christmas?'

'No, I haven't bought you a present because I didn't think you wanted anything.'

'Oh,' he said with a sigh.

'Have you bought me anything?' I asked.

'No,' he replied. 'I didn't think you wanted anything.'

'Right,' I said. 'Well that solves that.' He then told me he was thinking of buying me something. 'What's that?' I asked.

'I was thinking of buying you a walking stick,' he replied.

'What were you going to buy me a walking stick for? So I could wrap it around your neck?'

'No, it's not so you can wrap it around my neck. I've noticed you've been limping quite badly lately and I thought it might help you.'

'Well, what stopped you from buying me one then?'

He then looked me in the eyes and said, 'You'll know yourself when to buy one.'

A tear came to my eye and I told him, 'Let's hope I never have to buy one.'

'Yes,' he said, 'let's hope you don't.' And with that we decided to call it an early night – after all it was Christmas Eve.

I still wake up on Christmas Day morning feeling very excited, and this year was no different. Even though I am getting older now, I still like that feeling when you wake up and it's Christmas Day. The first thing I normally do is look at my hands and feet and say, 'Good morning, Uncle Arthur, and a very Merry Christmas to you.'

'Good morning and Happy Christmas to you,' he will reply. This year was no different, and so after we had given each other our Christmas greetings we got dressed and went downstairs.

Uncle Arthur suddenly made a beeline for the piano and asked if we could play a couple of tunes together.

'Like what?' I asked him.

'Why don't you play a couple of Christmas tunes?'

'Okay, I'll play you a couple of tunes, but only if you promise to leave me alone and let me reach the keys that I need to reach without giving me any grief.'

'I promise you,' he said. 'After all, it is Christmas Day.'

'Any requests?' I asked him.

'Yes,' he said, 'could you play "Jingle Bells"?'

'Of course I can play "Jingle Bells".' I pulled up my stool and proceeded to play "Jingle Bells", followed by a little bit of "White Christmas."'

When I finished, Uncle Arthur clapped and said, 'Well done, that was very nice. It's always nice to listen to someone tickling the ivories, especially on Christmas Day morning, because it gets the day off to a nice little start.'

And so with that, Christmas passed in the usual way: eating, drinking, watching telly, and the odd snowball fight. As the snow began to melt, in crept the New Year and a time to reflect. There is always a moment on New Year's Eve when I take a step back and think about the year that has just passed. I think about all the trials and tribulations that I have had with Uncle Arthur during the year. I think about all the really difficult times I have had with him and all the embarrassing moments that he has caused me, to the rare times when I have managed to cope with him and achieve something.

And so with that, the wild celebrations of New Year's Eve passed and a new year lay ahead.

When I woke up on that new January morning Uncle Arthur was there with me as usual, and my first thought was, I wonder what this year will bring for us both?

After saying our good mornings to each other I asked him if he was looking forward to anything in particular this year, and was there anything in particular he would like to do? He paused for a moment at my question and then said, 'Yes, there are a couple of things I would like.'

'Like what?' I asked. He told me that the first thing he wanted was a nice holiday in the sun. 'Why do you want a holiday in the sun?' I asked.

'Why not?' he answered.

So I said to him, 'You don't normally like me taking you on holiday to a warm place because when it's warm you can't be as grumpy or aggressive as you like to be with me.' He then said he would like me to go on holiday somewhere nice and warm because it would give me something to look forward to, and if I had something to look forward to I would be less grumpy myself. He was right, of course, another good way to overcome the bad days with Arthritis is to have something nice to look forward to, like a nice holiday in the sun. So I am hoping to grant Uncle Arthur his wish and maybe book a nice holiday for later this year.

'Is there anything else you'd like me to do for you this year?' I asked him.

'Yes, there is one thing,' he replied.

What he said next shocked me a little: 'Would you please stop calling me your Uncle Arthur and start calling me by my proper name.'

'But I've always called you my Uncle Arthur,' I told him.

'Yes, I know you have, but I prefer my common name of Arthritis.'

For the next few moments I thought about his request and then told him, 'Okay, I'll try my best to call you by your common name of Arthritis a bit more often than I do at the moment.'

He then paused and said, 'Thank you.'

Chapter Twelve

THE TRENCH

Over the weeks and months that were to follow, I would be forced to battle hard with my illness, because during these cold months of the year it is at its worst. Sometimes I would just feel like a soldier stuck in a muddy trench fighting my own war. You can liken fighting this disease to fighting a war because you will have so many battles with it, and some you will win and some you will lose.

On the occasions when you lose the battle, you must pull yourself up from that muddy trench and reload your rifle ready for the next battle, just like the soldier would do. Whenever you win a little battle with the illness, you must use that strength and triumph to carry on the fight. During our war with this illness we will be forced to fight hard day by day, night by night, week by week, month by month, and year by year. I always want to be like that soldier on the front line: brave and battle-hardened, but the simple fact is often I am not.

Sometimes I will just sit in the mud with my head between my knees and my rifle lying before me, not wanting to fight on. These are the worst times in my battle with the enemy. It will often take another lone soldier at my side to pick my rifle up, reload it for me and then pass it to me as though to say, Don't let the trumpets fade, son, don't give up the fight. What I am trying to say is that I am not in the trench alone, it is a trench of millions worldwide, and as we look out over the parapet of that muddy trench, we can see the battlefield, and on the other side of that battlefield is another trench, and dug deep into that trench is an enemy called Arthritis.

He is a very stubborn enemy, and we may have to fight him in the trenches and on the battlefields for many more years to come. Like the common soldier in the trench, he doesn't know when the war will end, and neither do the sufferers from Arthritis. The soldier will win his war when he sees the white flag of surrender, and we will win ours when a cure is found for this terrible illness.

Chapter Thirteen

A BRIEF SUMMARY

At this point a thought comes into my head: I've been rather rude because I haven't properly introduced myself. Well, my name is Dave, I am an ordinary working class chap with a rather ordinary life, and as yet have no wife and no children. I have a normal nine-to-five office job and I like the basic ordinary things in life and therefore class myself as, yes you guessed it, "ordinary".

It would be really nice to get married one day and start a family of my own, but I will just have to wait and see what happens on that front.

During this story I have mentioned my Uncle Arthur quite a lot as the story is about him, and in case you are wondering what his first name is, well I will tell you, it's "Psoriatic". His full name is Psoriatic Arthritis, and one of the reasons I call him Uncle Arthur is that Psoriatic Arthritis is quite a mouthful. I am not entirely sure where the name actually came from. He wasn't given it by some priest in a church, because he was never christened, and he was never christened because he has no parents. I think they probably disowned him when they realised what a horrible little problem child he was. I know he has a couple of distant cousins who go by the names of Osteo Arthritis and Rheumatoid Arthritis, and I have heard that they are even worse than my Uncle Arthur is, so I don't really want to meet them.

Basically Psoriatic Arthritis is just one of many forms of Arthritis.

If someone was to ask me what Arthritis is really like, I would simply tell them that it is like most illnesses: it will often bring you pain and discomfort and it will make you feel depressed and down in the dumps. But I would go on to say that each illness is different, and therefore the way in which we all cope with or fight the illnesses we have will be different, but in many ways the same, depending on the individual and the illness in question. Me personally, I would liken Arthritis to the Scarlet Pimpernel: it comes and goes when it pleases, but you never know when it is coming because it has many guises and therefore strikes you when you are not expecting it, and just like the Scarlet Pimpernel it is very cunning and clever, so be warned.

Chapter Fourteen

PRESENT DAY

We come to the present day, and I am writing the last part of my story. I am sitting on a grass bank by the river, the sun is out and there is a lovely breeze. I am listening to the calming sound of the water, and I can hear the birds singing in the distance. It's a place where I often come to relax and gather my thoughts because it's so peaceful and quiet.

In case you are wondering where my Uncle Arthur is, well, he is sitting here with me, and of late I have really been struggling with him. It saddens me to tell you that there are now some mornings when I struggle even to dress myself without being in pain, because he has decided to move into most parts of my body, which is quite depressing. He seems to have just got worse and worse since the Marathon and because of that I am now being forced to give him some of his favourite tablets in the hope of keeping him quiet. Maybe he has never forgiven me for finishing the Marathon, and maybe this is payback time? He knows that the One Thousand Six Hundred and Fifty Pounds I raised (thanks to all the kind people that sponsored me for the Marathon) will go a long way in the bid to rid society of this horrible disease.

Even though I am struggling at the moment with my Arthritis, today I feel really at peace with myself. My story is just one person's journey with this illness, and I know there are many more like me, and as I am sitting here wondering what to write next, a smile comes to my face, because I am realising that there is no real ending to my story. Because there can't be: there can't be an ending until a cure is found for Arthritis. I must enjoy the feelings and thoughts I have today because I know tomorrow could be different. I know deep down that nothing is going to change with me and Uncle Arthur in the near future, but I have to live in hope that one day he will walk out of my life forever. I dream of the day when I am standing looking down at his grave: I will celebrate the day he dies and leaves innocent people to live their lives in peace.

His headstone will probably read something like:

David Smalley

Here lies Arthritis
Died peacefully after causing pain,
grief and sadness
to many people for many years.
Never loved, Never missed, and Never will be.

When he dies he will never lie in a place where people can visit him, he will never have fresh flowers put upon his grave. He will lie in a place where the leaves from the trees will never fall on him, and where the birds will never sing to him. Let us all wish for that day. As for me, I will carry on the journey with my Arthritis, trying my best to battle on through the bad days, and smiling through the good days. As for today, I only have one thing left to say to my Uncle Arthur: 'Die, you bastard, just die ...'